# Simple keto cookbook:

*An Effective Approach to Keto Lifestyle, with Everyday Low-Carb Recipes*

The information in the following pages is broadly considered to be a truthful and accurate account of facts and as such any inattention, use or misuse of the information in question by the reader will render any resulting actions solely under their purview. There are no scenarios in which the publisher or the original author of this work can be in any fashion deemed liable for any hardship or damages that may befall them after undertaking information described herein.

Additionally, the information in the following pages is intended only for informational purposes and should thus be thought of as universal. As befitting its nature, it is presented without assurance regarding its prolonged validity or interim quality. Trademarks that are mentioned are done without written consent and can in no way be considered an endorsement from the trademark holder.

# Introduction

Congratulations on buying *Simple Keto Cookbook,* and thank you for doing so.

The following chapters will tell the story of Elena, a 28-year-old woman who has decided to embark on a healthier lifestyle. The first step of that journey is to find the right diet plan and begin to lose weight.

With her sister getting married in June, Elena can't help but feel a time crunch on looking and feeling her best. She will explore diet options, discovering diet trends that are not successful and learning why the ketogenic diet is. Elena's friend Janet will help outline how to implement ketosis into your diet properly and how to keep the weight off once you reach your goal!

While following Elena's progress, we will learn how to compile a ketogenic meal plan, tips and tricks for successful grocery shopping, and how to build a more active and healthy routine. We will also learn about possible side effects of the ketogenic diet and how to manage them.

Of course, this book should not take the place of medical advice from your doctor. Although the diet is safe, you should always consult your physician before making any major dietary changes in case you have a condition that might create unforeseen obstacles. With that said, you will be hard-pressed to find a more in-depth or easy to understand book on ketosis out there.

There are plenty of books on this subject on the market, thanks again for choosing this one! Every effort was made to ensure it is full of as much useful information as possible, please enjoy!

# Chapter 1: Meet Elena

Elena couldn't pretend she wasn't expecting the news. Her sister, Charlotte, had been seeing Tim for almost two years. Everyone knew he'd propose, eventually.

Still, when Elena received the text message on her way to work that Charlotte and Tim had set a date, she couldn't help but feel her anxiety build. Three years ago, Elena moved away from her hometown, and she hadn't been back since. In the time she'd been gone, she had gained thirty pounds. Through careful angling of her Facebook photos, she had managed to keep any of her back home friends from knowing about her drastic weight gain.

Now, with an unavoidable trip home only months away, Elena knew it was time to get serious about dropping the weight. Fortunately, Elena was young- only 28- and did not have any dietary issues or health problems that would prohibit her from getting busy on dropping those pounds

When Elena arrived at her office, she couldn't get her mind off of setting a new goal for a healthier lifestyle. During slow periods at work, she found herself surfing the internet for diet tips and exercise routines.

It seemed like every site Elena stumbled on was trying to sell her a product that promised to burn her fat in under a week, a wrap that would tighten her skin and dissolve the fat from the outside in, or a new method of meditation that would somehow trick her metabolism into speeding up.

Elena was not convinced. When lunchtime arrived, her co-worker, Janet, asked her if she would like to join her lunch at a nearby grille. Elena was hungry but was not in the mood to eat.

"I'd love to," Elena explained. "Unfortunately, I just found out this morning that my sister is getting married this summer. I need to lose weight before the wedding, and I'm not sure eating out is a great idea today."

Janet chuckled. "Come with me," she coaxed. "I want to tell you about ketosis. I've been in your shoes. Before you met me, I, too, was in need of a healthier diet. I shed forty pounds just by changing what I eat, and I didn't have to starve!"

Elena was skeptical, but without any other options, she decided to go along with Janet and find out what this ketogenic diet was all about.

# Chapter 2: What is the Keto Diet?

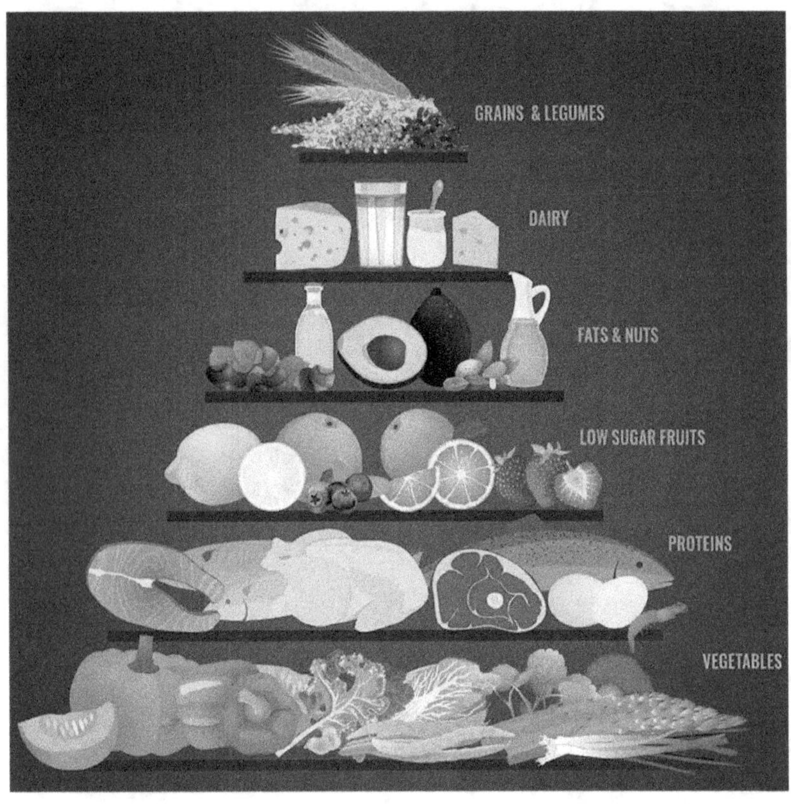


When the ladies arrived at the restaurant, Elena was still confused by Janet's use of the term "ketosis," and how a person could possibly not worry about calories and still lose weight.

She decided to observe Janet's eating habits as well as listen to what she had to say.

Janet did not even open her menu. She already knew what she wanted to order, so Elena decided to order the same to see if the keto diet plan was really all Janet was building it up to be. When the waiter came to the table, Janet ordered water to drink, a medium rare 8 oz. steak and a side salad with balsamic dressing. Elena was pleased with the order. It was far better than anything she would have chosen for herself, anyway.

"So, how does this actually work?" Elena asked. "Even as I sit here, I'm absolutely horrified that I don't know how many calories this steak is." Janet laughed. "Let me explain," she said.

Over the next thirty minutes, Janet outlined the keto diet as follows:
The body typically burns carbohydrates, or carbs, for energy. When the body achieves ketosis, though, it begins to burn ketones from the liver, instead. The purpose of achieving ketosis is to stop taking in carbs, which can have other harmful effects on the body.

Carbs create glucose and insulin. Glucose is a molecule built mostly from sugar, which is often produced to burn for energy. Insulin is produced to process glucose.

The problem with burning glucose is that your body fat is not needed for any purpose, and it is then stored. When we reduce the amount of carbohydrates we consume and instead boost our fat and protein intake, the body enters ketosis.
"How do I know if I'm in ketosis, though?" Elena asked. She was intrigued by the idea of this diet but couldn't wrap her head around how you can change the entire way your body works, simply by altering what you eat.

"It's actually quite simple," Janet said. "Anyone can enter ketosis, just by following a few simple steps."

She continued her explanation:

Ketosis is achieved when we deprive our bodies of carbohydrates, not calories. The body will begin to look for new fuel to burn for energy. When it does, it will begin to produce ketones from the fatty deposits stored in the liver. The human body is very adaptive. When we overload ourselves with fats and take away carbohydrates, the body will see the fats as a new source of energy, not only burning the fat we take in, but also pulling fat from the body.

Because of the way people tend to eat, our bodies have become used to the process of breaking down carbs and burning them. Inside each of us, we have an army of enzymes that have been developed solely for carb break down. Most of our bodies, though, don't have many enzymes produced to break down fats. This is why so many of us find that, despite counting calories, we are constantly storing fats in our system.

As our bodies learn to break down fats in ketosis, we will use up the rest of our glucose. Soon, we will have very little excess glucose distributed throughout our bodies, which means fat will stop being deposited and will, instead, begin depleting.

There are a few simple steps that need to be followed to achieve ketosis:

1. Limit the amount of carbohydrates you are taking in. Most people count only the net carbs of thcir food. With the keto diet, you must focus on total carbs. It is important not to take in more than 35 total carbs in a single day.

2. Eat plenty of protein, but don't go overboard. Too much protein can cause ketosis to slow. If you are trying to lose weight, it is recommended to stay at about 0.8 grams of protein per pound of lean body mass each day. Lean body mass is a calculation that determines your total body weight minus the weight of your body fat. In simplified terms, it is a few pounds under your ideal body weight.

3. Drink plenty of water. Most people see best results in ketosis when they drink a full gallon of water a day. Water helps the body function and also is great at suppressing appetite throughout the day. Try to spread your water intake evenly throughout the day, so you aren't over hydrating at the end of the day to reach your gallon goal.

4. Don't worry about the fat you eat. Fat is the primary source of energy on the keto diet, so make sure you are always getting enough of it. You don't lose weight on the keto diet by starving yourself. Instead, you lose weight by changing how your body works.

5. Try to limit your snacking. Again, you shouldn't feel hungry while on the keto diet, so it's okay to have snacks planned. However, you should avoid eating those snacks if you don't absolutely need them. Planning snacks will keep you from binging on something unhealthy out of hunger, but don't feel like you have to eat the snack just because you have planned for it. Instead, plan a cook- and- prep free snack that you can simply ignore if you aren't in need of stifling your hunger.

6. Work slowly into exercise. Exercise makes us hungry, which should be avoided in the early days of ketosis. Try a 20 or 30-minute walk per day until you make it through the ketosis barrier, then you can slowly add to your exercise regimen over time.

7. Stop drinking soda and other sugary beverages. A large percentage of the carbs we take in come from soda and sugared drink consumption. We often overlook the carbs we take in from drinks because we don't think of them as food. Quitting soda will give you a huge jump in limiting

your daily carb intake. Besides, there are simply far better ways to stay hydrated.

"Wait a minute," Elena interrupted. "So, I understand how the keto diet works to burn fat, but can it really be healthy if it completely changes how the body functions? The body does more than take in and burn food. How do I know I'm not damaging the rest of my body by jumping into this?"

Janet smiled. "You'd be surprised," she said. "The keto diet provides some benefits for the body that go far beyond just burning fat."

With that, she began outlining the other benefits of the keto diet:

1. The keto diet controls blood sugar. Because you are taking in less carbs, your body is not producing as much glucose. This makes the keto diet an exemplary diet idea for those that are at risk of developing diabetes. As your body learn to function without the high glucose levels, it will produce less of them, which keeps blood sugar levels and insulin levels in check.

2. It can improve mental focus. Many people who are on the keto diet are on it simply to improve mental focus. Ketones are the best fuel our body can produce for brain function. When we lower our carb intake and avoid spikes in glucose and insulin, this helps our brain focus and concentrate on other tasks. Additionally, fatty acids break down into great enzymes that benefit the functions of the brain.

3. You will have more energy and be less hungry. When your body is burning a more reliable source of energy, it will keep you feeling energized throughout the day. Fats are the most effective source of fuel for energy that there is! Additionally, a fatty diet is more satisfying and leaves the body feeling satisfied longer. You won't feel nearly as hungry on a keto diet as you would through calorie counting or other means of dieting.

4. The keto diet has been proven to help control seizure disorders. In fact, the keto diet was developed in the 1920s to treat epilepsy in children. It is still a widely

used method of seizure control in kids because it enables the body to work to control seizures without taking in a lot of medications, which have not been widely studied in terms of effects on young people, just yet.

5.  It will give you clearer skin. Do you remember being an awkward high schooler with acne? Were you ever told that your skin broke out because you were eating too much sugar? Well, as it turns out, that's not an old wives' tale. Carbohydrates do contribute significantly to skin breakouts. When we take in fewer carbs, our body produced less glucose. Without the glucose, your skin will become more clear.

6.  The keto diet stabilizes cholesterol and blood pressure levels. Your body's triglyceride levels are improved when you are taking in fewer carbs. This prevents buildup in your arteries and keeps your blood pumping at a manageable level, optimizing you to stay energized all day long without over-exerting yourself.

"I have to admit, this all sounds way too good to be true," Elena says. "Are you sure there aren't any risks?"

"There are risks with any diet," Janet explains. "You should definitely always speak to your physician before beginning any new diet plan. If you are already diabetic, the keto diet might not be the answer you're looking for. You also should be careful that you aren't suffering from any kidney disease or blood disorders before beginning the keto diet. Also, with any diet, it's important not to become weight- obsessed. Most eating disorders begin during otherwise healthy diet plans.

Speak to your physician and make sure this is the right plan for you. That also adds an extra person to your team to keep an eye on your progress and ensure you aren't going overboard. Losing weight is always a good feeling, but it shouldn't be done without the added goal of developing better lifestyle habits. With everything, you have to find a balance that works for you."

When Elena returned to the office, she took a moment before resuming her work to schedule an appointment with her doctor.

# Chapter 3:
# How to Compile
# a Meal Plan

After getting approval from her doctor, Elena was excited to begin her new keto diet. She decided the first step in the process was meal planning.
She began researching tips for how to plan her meals online but was- again- overwhelmed with information she didn't need. She decided, instead, she would create her own method.

After all, the most important part of planning meals is to understand that everyone is different. What works for one person might not work for the next. Some of us have busy families. Some of us live alone.

The most important part of preparing your meal plan is to make sure the timing works for you.

Elena decided to plan her meals for two weeks, prepping what she could ahead of time and doing the bulk of her weekly cooking on

Sundays, when she was usually at home all day, anyway, and on Wednesday afternoons, which she typically devoted to computer games, since none of her regular television shows were on that night.

Meal planning is really that simple for all of us. We all have our own routines, but we can usually find time to add in a new task that will be healthy and beneficial for us.

Before beginning her keto diet, Elena took a few days to research recipes. She wanted to make sure she found recipes that worked for her, nutritionally, fit her tastes, and were things she would enjoy preparing. At times, she felt like she was being indulgent, but she knew it was all for the best- she was learning how to maintain a healthier lifestyle!

By researching her recipes and organizing a meal plan for two weeks ahead of time, she was avoiding last-minute decisions about what- or where- to eat. This would keep her from making unhealthy choices in the beginning days of her diet. It would also help her expand her horizons in terms of how she would meal plan throughout the future.

She scoured the internet for recipes she would enjoy, looked at some of her grandmother's old cookbooks, and paid close attention to ingredients. When she wasn't sure about the nutritional makeup of a certain ingredient, she took the time to research it. As she planned her recipes, she used an online calculator to determine their carb, fat, and protein content and made note of each along with the recipes she chose. This helped her figure out which recipes she could pair together to ensure she didn't cross her daily threshold.

Elena chose to type her recipes into a word processor, printing her own two- week meal plan and cookbook at the beginning of the week. This not only kept her recipes well organized and easy to read, but it made compiling her grocery list easier, as well.

Elena checked her calendar for any upcoming events or plans that she might have to alter her diet around. She and her friends typically get together a few nights a week to watch some of their favorite shows. Knowing this, Elena planned to prepare enough to feed her friends on these nights, and to prepare foods that she knew they would enjoy.

Elena also knows she's a comfort eater. She tends to want to grill out or eat a more ethnic or spicy food when the weather is nice and have something heavy and warm when the weather is chilly. She looked at her extended weather forecast to determine what days would be optimal for grilling and which days she would prefer to have something heavier, like a nice bowl of stew or a hearty casserole.

Once Elena had a good idea of which recipes she wanted to use, she started a calendar. She decided to start a separate Google calendar just for her meal plan. This way, she would be able to easily swap recipes if other things came up, and she would be able to check from her phone to remind herself what was on the menu if she began wondering while working. It also helped her to visualize the meal plan to maintain a sense of control over what meals she paired with each other to give herself better control over her own carb counting and diet experience as a whole.

Next, Elena decided to choose a day to devote to her shopping. Typically, Elena orders in her groceries, but she knew that she would need to do her own selecting to feel connected to what she was going to eat. She wanted to be able to check freshness and labels on her own. She decided to devote the following Saturday entirely to her shopping trip.

In Elena's research, she wound up with away more recipes than she needed. She decided to check her local grocery ads for sales to determine which recipes would be the best. She found that her local market had a sale on chicken breasts and avocados. She decided to pick recipes that used these two ingredients over others that would be more expensive. She placed the extra recipes in a folder to be used in her next recipe rotation.

Because Elena lives alone and so many of her recipes are compiled for the purpose of multiple servings, she purchased freezer bags and containers to help her store away excess servings to be used in future meal plan rotations. This would not only help her budget future grocery trips but would also prevent food waste and save time in later days.

Elena created a spreadsheet for her groceries, then began sorting through her selected recipes, tallying her needed groceries. Because of the spreadsheet, she was able to easily edit her list to include additional quantities of certain groceries as her recipes called for them. Once she had her grocery list complete, she organized it into separate headings to help her find the items in the store in an organized fashion.

With her meal plan and grocery list both successfully compiled, Elena was ready to begin shopping.

# Chapter 4: Surviving the Grocery Store

On Saturday, when Elena was finally ready to do her grocery shopping, she looked back over her list one final time with dread. Grocery shopping is no fun for Elena. She has never liked the chore of fighting the grocery store crowd to gather items for the week. This is one of the reasons Elena has put on weight.

Similarly, groceries are expensive. When Elena looked at her compiled grocery list, she felt her stomach twist into a knot of dread. It seems less expensive to drop $10 here or there on a fast, convenient meal. Dropping a lot of money all at once can feel like a kick to teeth. Elena resolved to go into the task with an open mind, knowing that it was worth the time and short-term investment to better her health.

For many, it's easier to buy fast food or other convenience meals than it is to deal with a dreaded grocery store trip. Thankfully, Elena had spoken with several of her friends and family members and learned their tips and tricks for easy grocery shopping:

1. Eat first. A lot of people make the mistake of going to the grocery store on an empty stomach. When you do this, you put yourself at risk of purchasing things because they look good, rather than buying things you need. You'll end up spending more money and not getting the things that are good for you. Elena helped herself to one final meal out before beginning her keto diet. She chose her favorite restaurant and ordered her favorite dish. This was her way of saying goodbye to the unhealthy habit of convenience food, and it also helped her feel satisfied before facing the piles of groceries at the nearby store..

2. If you're used to eating out, look back at your bank activity and do a running tally. Totaling up the amount of money you have spent throughout the month on eating out, small grocery trips or other foods can put into perspective how much money you will now save by preparing foods at home. Sometimes we don't

realize how much money we spend on food because we are doing it in small quantities. Making one large grocery trip, while it will seem like a lot of money to drop all at once, will actually likely be less expensive at the end of the month than your usual style of eating.

3. Stick to your menu. It can be easy, when shopping, to see a different food item you want to try in place of what you have already planned to buy. This is a slippery slope to forsaking the list, entirely. Instead of trying to swap it into this trip for a currently planned recipe, make a note to include it in your next meal plan.

4. Make your list ahead of time. Elena has already completed this important step, so she's good to go. To review, though, having a complete and organized list means you won't forget ingredients or get frustrated with your experience and leave. When we leave the store, we inevitably must return. In doing so, we open ourselves up to lots of potential impulse purchases, which puts our diet at risk.

5. Do a running tally and stick to your budget. Estimate the cost of your groceries ahead of time, so you aren't suckered with sticker shock at the check out aisle. Always round up when in doubt, and remind yourself throughout your shopping trip to not take on extra groceries or else you risk overextending your budget.

6. Carry a calculator. Don't be duped into thinking that larger quantity purchases are always cheaper. Do the math- you will sometimes find that, even when a box advertises "10 percent free," or other such jargon, you are actually still paying for the difference. Similarly, conveniently packaged products are sometimes more expensive to buy than those you will need to separate and package yourself. If you are trying to pinch pennies, the added time spent working out the price per ounce might well be worth the savings you'll uncover.

7. Coupons are worth the effort. It might seem like a laughable pastime, but the savings really can add up. Just make sure

you aren't purchasing items that are on sale just because they're on sale. Skim the newspaper inserts for coupons that apply to your grocery list and clip those. The rest can be stored in an envelope to look through later. If you are extra organized, you can keep separate envelopes sorted by due date. This will ensure you don't become the nuisance in the check out aisle trying to pass an expired coupon.

8. Don't be frustrated by out-of-stock sale items. Instead, find a manager and ask for a rain check. It's worth coming back later in the week for the needed items, especially if you need a lot of them!

9. Don't be afraid of store brands. Often, we find ourselves stuck in a false way of thinking that generic brand groceries are somehow nutritionally sub-par to name brand. Not only is this not true, but it is often the opposite. Check the nutrition labels and compare the store brand item and the name brand. Name brands often have added ingredients for longer preservation and slight boosts in flavor. You probably won't even notice the

difference, taste-wise, but you will potentially save money and keep certain chemicals out of your body by going for the cheaper, less fancy label.

10.  Watch the register. Human error happens. Sometimes, store sales aren't entered properly into the computer system. Don't be afraid to speak up if you are being overcharged for something.

11. Go during a slow time of the day. Elena decided to do her grocery shopping later in the evening on Saturday because she knows most people are out enjoying their weekend at that time. She was pleased to find that the grocery store was not overly crowded or busy and the weekend stockers were hard at work replenishing the produce supply. As she shopped, she realized that it would be worth the savings to come back early the next morning for meat, when the meat department marked down the prior day's meat supply. Several of the items she intended to purchase was in stock Saturday evening, which meant they

would likely still be in stock on Sunday morning at a fraction of the cost.

12. Buy as "clean" as possible. Processed foods are full of additives that will work against you in dieting. Buy things as close to their natural form as possible to maximize weight loss potential and improve your overall health.

13. Clean out your fridge and pantry before you go. You'll need places to pack the groceries away. Getting rid of old leftovers and grocery items that have expired will not only clear space but will give you an opportunity to take inventory of any supplies you already have on hand. Crossing these items off of your list will decrease your overall spending.

14. Become a store savings card holder. Many grocery stores allow you to rack up points with memberships. These points can often be used for savings on future grocery trips, free items, or savings at the gas pump. As you begin to prepare more meals at home, you will find it worth the

15. Skip the beverage aisle. Again, soda and other sweetened drinks are full of carbohydrates, preservatives, and other ingredients that are simply not good for you. The average daily soda drinker spends nearly $3,000 a year on carbonated beverages alone! Not only will you cut back your carb intake, but you'll also put money back into your grocery budget.

Using these tips, Elena's trip to the store proved to be a breeze! She was pleasantly surprised by the stress, time, and money saved. When she returned home, she began prepping her food for the week. She washed and dried her vegetables, chopped her onions, and pre-cooked any ingredients she could to save time. She stacked her containers of pre-prepped ingredients neatly into her fridge for easy access and then took on the task of cleaning up her kitchen.

Yes, food prep is messy and time-consuming, but Elena was comforted, when the work was done, with the knowledge that she was heading into her week with the hard part of her meal preparation already behind her.

Next, Elena knew that she would need to develop a slowly- building exercise routine that would fit in well with her work schedule, her physical activity level, and with her new keto diet.

Before we get to that point, though, here are some food prep tips you can implement in your own kitchen:

1. Cook a whole week in a day. One of the biggest and most common mistakes busy people make is waiting until the last minute to start dinner. That leads to giving up on the idea of cooking, a run for fast food, and all around unhealthy choices. We can't predict bad days. A tough day at the office, bad traffic on the way home, a disagreement with a friend, or even something as simple as a headache can cause us to feel out of the mood to cook when the time comes to prepare the healthy meal we have planned.

We can avoid this by completing the meal earlier in the week, then freezing it to be reheated on the day we intend to eat it. If a week's worth of meals seems like too much, at least do a few days at a time. You'll thank yourself later.

2. It doesn't have to be complicated. You aren't on a cooking competition show. Nobody is grading you on how exotic or full your meal is. If you are looking for a recipe and feel like you're back in Chemistry class, don't feel bad about setting that one to the side and choosing something different for your meal plan. Nobody expects five stars from you.

3. If you can afford it, splurge on pre-cut produce. This will save you tons of time when it comes to pre-packaging your ingredients.

4. Cook a bunch of chicken at once. If most of your recipes are calling for shredded chicken, there's no shame in loading the crock pot with chicken breasts, shredding, and bagging for later. You can boil chicken and save the broth. You can

cook a whole chicken and use separate cuts for different meals. Rotisserie chicken, baked chicken, and roasted chicken are versatile recipe staples.

5.  Buy clear food storage containers. Portioning your meals, ingredients, and snacks before you need them saves time and helps you eat less. When you store them in clear containers, you don't have to guess. You can find what you're needing exactly when you need it.

6.  Pre-bag smoothie ingredients. If, like Elena, you find that smoothies are the quickest breakfast solution at your disposal, pre-make your smoothie bags, then move the next morning's bag from the freezer to the fridge the night before you need it. This will thaw it to a blendable consistency and save you time from measuring in the morning. Even milk and yogurt can be portioned into ice trays and frozen ahead!

7.  Prep immediately. You won't feel like pulling everything out to prep later. Save yourself time and trouble by prepping

right away and clearing the entirety of the mess in one fell swoop.

8. Keep your fridge well organized. Knowing what you have is half the battle of knowing what you need when grocery day comes. Label your shelves and let everything have its designated place. Soon, you'll be taking inventory without much more than a glance.

9. Make big batches. You might only need pasta sauce once this week, but there's little point in measuring exact ingredients for one serving. Make a whole pot and freeze the excess. It will save you time next week.

10.     Finally, don't prep too far out. Remember, food will spoil. You need to be conscious of how long your meals can keep before they will need to be thrown away.

# Chapter 5: Building a Work-Out Routine that Works Out

Elena knows that one of the riskiest parts of developing a new workout routine is realizing that going in too enthusiastically and overexerting herself might make her less likely to stick to the routine long term. As a result, she starts by gathering information on resources in her community that might be helpful to her and taking an inventory of her current physical activity limitations.

When we are out of shape, we can't do as much. We shouldn't expect to be able to do a full workout in the first weeks of our routine when our body is only beginning to adjust to a healthier lifestyle. This is especially vital to remember when your body is going through ketosis.

Developing your own work out routine should be done with consideration for your biology, age, goals, health conditions, and the amount of free time and resources you have available to you. Some people live in metropolitan areas where gyms are available close by. Others live in more rural surroundings where public gyms are few and far between. Perhaps your apartment building has a swimming pool and a workout room you can use for free. Perhaps you don't have any of these at your disposal or can't afford a gym membership.

The good news is that a workout routine can be developed for anyone, regardless of physical, geographical, time, or financial limitations. Because Elena' schedule often varies, she decided to use a variety of work out types to plan her routine.

Developing a workout routine for yourself can seem equally daunting to creating a meal plan and shopping list, but don't worry. There are just a few basic points you need to keep in mind when doing so:

1. Is it going to work? Have realistic expectations. If you work forty hours a week, volunteer twenty, and go home to a busy family, you probably won't find time to devote an hour a day at the gym. Similarly, if you are currently twice your

ideal body weight, you probably won't be doing three mile runs anytime soon. Don't be so hard on yourself or so enthusiastic about the weight loss that you sabotage yourself with unrealistic expectations fresh out the gate.

2. Are you safe? Again, consider your current physical limitations. You can always increase the difficulty of your workout later. Don't let yourself become injured or dehydrate because you are trying to overdo it. Instead, pace yourself and build as you go. By the same token, don't swim in water that is too deep for you. Don't walk your mile in unsafe territory. Don't ignore safety protocol at the gym.

3. Are you having fun? Of course, exercise won't be a party, but it shouldn't be something that you dread, either. If you find yourself despising the idea of working out, you need to change something. If you aren't enjoying yourself, you're setting yourself up to quit.

With this in mind, Elena made a list of exercises she would enjoy trying and then looked up the health benefits of each. Using this information, she figured out which exercises would be the most beneficial for her starting out and made a list of exercises that would be better implemented at a later date, when she was more physically fit and could safely begin expanding her routine.

Next, Elena made a list of places she could work out. She has a gym available in her apartment complex, as well as a pool. She also lives in a fairly safe community with ample parks and bike trails, where long distance walking would be tolerable and without added risk.

Finally, she looked at her schedule and made a list of times that would work for her to implement her exercises.

Elena knows she has half an hour every morning to devote to an exercise routine and different amounts of time available in the evenings, depending on the day. Elena decides to start her routine by first utilizing the morning time slot, then add more evening routines in later as her tolerance for physical activity improved.

Elena decided to target a different part of her body each day of the week and give herself weekends off, at first.

Her beginning routine looked like this:

| Monday Morning | Squats to target the Quads |
|---|---|
| Tuesday Morning | Push-ups to target the chest, shoulders, and triceps |
| Wednesday Morning | Pull-ups to target the back, biceps, and forearms |
| Thursday Morning | Step Ups to target the butt and hamstrings. |
| Friday Morning | Exercise ball crunches to target the abs and lower back. |

Elena also found a body stretch routine to implement before beginning her exercise sets each morning.

The stretch routine went as follows:

1. The Marathon Stretch: Step forward with your right foot and lower into a lunge. Place your fingertips on the floor or on a

firm cushion if you can't reach the floor.
Breathe in, then exhale as you strengthen
your right leg. Return, slowly, to the
lunge position and repeat four times
before switching sides.

2.  The Side Stretch: Stand up tall with your
    feet touching and your arms extended
    over your head. Clasp your hands tightly
    together, interlacing your fingers except
    for the pointer fingers, which should
    remain extended. Inhale as you reach
    upward as high as you can. Breathe out as
    you bend your upper body to the right
    and take five slow breaths. Slowly return
    to an upright position, then repeat on
    your left side.

3.  Hang Forward: Stand up tall with your
    feet spaced at the hips. Slightly bend your
    knees and interlace your fingers behind
    your back. You can hold a dishtowel
    behind your back if your arms can't
    reach. Take a deep breath in and
    straighten your arms, which will extend
    your chest. Exhale and bend forward at
    the waist, letting your hands stretch up
    toward your head and hold for five
    breaths.

4.  Low Arch: Step your right foot forward into a lunge position and lower your left knee to the floor. Bring your arms to the front of your right leg and hook your thumbs together with your palms pointed at the floor. Breathe in as you sweep your arms overhead, stretching as far back as is comfortable. Take five deep breaths and then switch sides.

5.  Sit on the floor with your legs straight in front of you. Bend your right knee and step your right foot over the left leg. Put your right hand down on the floor to support you with your fingers extended. Bend your left elbow and turn to your right, putting the back of your arm against your center. Sit up tall and inhale deep, then exhale slowly. As you exhale, twist your body and press your arm into your leg while you look over your shoulder. Slowly return to the center. Do this three times, then switch sides.

6.  Remain seated on the floor and straighten your legs back out in front of you. Bring the soles of your feet together and let your knees drop to the ground.

Hold your shins as you inhale and stretch your body upward, chest first. Exhale and hinge forward at the hips without bending and put your hands, palms down, on the ground in front of you. Hold this for five slow breaths.

After doing her stretches, Elena would feel better as she moved into her daily morning routine. She started slow with three sets of her exercise each day. Her second week, she upped it to four sets a day. By week three, she was doing five sets of her morning exercise every day.

Before long, she was able to introduce an afternoon workout, as well. By doing the proper stretches, she decreased her risk of being sore from her new workout routine, which increased her likelihood of maintaining it long- term.

Elena went back to her list of resources and exercises she would like to try. She also looked at her time available for exercise.

Elena had learned in her research that muscle is actually not built during exercise. Instead, muscle gets broken down during exercise and then rebuilds stronger during resting. She knew that balancing workouts with rest would help

her gain muscle mass, which would make her stronger and healthier overall.
Elena also knew that cardio workouts are the best for losing weight.

The more Elena researched, the more she learned about how exercise works. For example:

1.  Just because you exercise doesn't mean it's okay to sit a majority of the rest of your time. Sitting all day can put you at risk of heart disease and diabetes, even if you are otherwise physically active. Moving more often throughout the day will help your body from feeling sedentary, which can improve your overall health. Even if you are simply spending fifteen minutes a few times a day to take a quick walk up and down the office steps, it's crucial that you get in time on your feet.

2.  You don't get thin because you exercise. Dietary changes make up for 80 percent of weight loss. Exercise is an added bonus that improves your overall health, but how and what you eat will make much

more difference in the long run where the scale is concerned.

3.  Stretching isn't good if you plan to run. Stretching can actually decrease your efficiency when it comes to running because your body can be too limber. While stretching is important for all other forms of workouts, you should skip it if you're putting on your running shoes. Instead, warm up with a half mile walk.

4.  Achieving fitness goals helps you achieve life goals. A healthy lifestyle helps people achieve and maintain the discipline required to achieve the other goals they set in their lives. A study in the Archives of Internal Medicine has even revealed that smokers and drinkers are twice likely to quit and stay toxin free if they exercise than those who don't.

5.  Statistically, women are weaker today than they used to be. This is contributed to a growing stress women are putting on themselves to be thin, rather than strong. It has become a new belief in society that muscles are not attractive to women, so

rather than developing healthy exercise routines, women are simply starving their bodies of calories. While the "waif" look might be visually appealing by fashionable standards, having poor muscle make up can severely impact a woman's health. Muscle weakness is contributed to back and joint pain, osteoporosis, and even pregnancy loss.

6. Married couples exercise less. The Department of Health completed a poll that found only about a quarter of all married couples questioned were completing regular exercise routines. This is contributed to some factors including the busier lifestyle of becoming parents, insecurity about exercising together, and that married people sometimes become complacent about their health and appearance as they grow more comfortable with one another.

7. Social Media is actually good for fitness motivation. Recent studies show that being afraid of having someone tag us in an unflattering photo is a huge contributing factor to many of us living

healthier lifestyles. Fitbit confirmed these findings when they identified that unflattering Facebook photos were the number one weight loss trigger for men and women between the ages of 20 and 30 in the United Kingdom. Additionally, when our friends show off their fitness brags, we feel motivated to complete and post some of our own.

Equipped with all her new knowledge about exercise and building a fitness routine, Elena organized one of her own.

In the end, it looked like this:

| | |
|---|---|
| Monday Morning | Squats to target the Quads |
| Monday Evening | Thirty minutes in the pool. |
| Tuesday Morning | Push-ups to target the chest, shoulders, and triceps |
| Tuesday Evening | Two-mile walk at the local park. |
| Wednesday Morning | Pull-ups to target the back, biceps, and forearms |
| Wednesday Evening | Yoga class at the local studio. |
| Thursday Morning | Step Ups to target the butt and hamstrings. |
| Thursday Evening | Ride a bike to and from work, since Thursday evenings are otherwise busy. |
| Friday Morning | Exercise ball crunches to target the abs and lower back. |
| Friday Evening | Fifteen-minute cycles on the machines in the apartment complex gym. |

Eventually, Elena found that she felt better than she had in years. Because she was ready to take on more, she joined her local Roller Derby team, adding an additional workout to her Saturday!

As you explore your own work out routines, keep in mind that you can always add more later. It is always better to start off slow. You don't even have to start with a daily work out. In fact, many find that working out two or three times a week at first is plenty.

As your body begins to feel stronger, you can add one or two workouts a week until you have built a workout regimen that will not only challenge you but that you can also maintain. Be sure to do exercises that are not only beneficial for you but are also enjoyable.

Remember exercise doesn't have to be like boot camp. Take your dog for a walk in a place where there is pretty scenery. Go swimming with your family. Play a game of kickball with the kids.

As long as you are up and moving and burning energy, you are already succeeding at working out.

Here are a few more tips and tricks you can use to make your work out more enjoyable:

1. Enlist a friend for comradery. Maybe you have a friend that is also always talking about trying to get healthier. Reach out to them and see if they want to join you on your journey. Exercise isn't always fun to do when you're by yourself. Find a friend that can come along for the added benefit of a hang out day. This will also help you be more accountable. Everyone wants to skip a workout, but nobody wants to bail on a friend.

2. Create a special work out playlist. There's no reason why you should have to work out in silence. Compile a list of your favorite songs and let the music move you! Workouts are meant for silly energy. Fast-paced, fun music will always motivate you to keep your body in motion.

3. Check for local class offerings. Don't let yourself feel cheese balled by the old notion that group fitness is all spandex

and sweatbands, sweating over vintage pop. Exercise classes have come a long way in recent years. With the inception of indoor surfing, rock climbing, kickboxing, and the take-off of other novelty sports, people are moving and building strength and stamina in ways they never thought they could.

4.  Don't watch the clock. Just enjoy yourself. A watched pot never boils, and a watched clock doesn't burn calories. Just get into what you are doing and the time will pass before you know it.

5.  Pretend you're in a game- or actually be in one! Exergaming is a new craze in the video world and fitness world where high tech games suck you in and award points and level ups for physical activity. Play till your heart's content and burn off energy while you're doing it.

6.  Be a philanthropist. There are tons of walking and work out apps that will reward your hard work with donations to your favorite charities. Do a quick search and see what's available in your area. You

can be rewarded for how fast you run a mile, how many consecutive days you check into your local gym, or even how far you walk your dog (or a virtual dog)! Better yourself and better the world!

7. Start with the worst and work to the best. The hardest part of your exercise routine should be thrown out of the way early on so you can enjoy the decline to the more fun parts of the activity.

8. Bet on it. Find someone else who is trying to maintain a healthier lifestyle. Place bets on each other's progress and get competitive. You don't have to gamble money. It can be something as simple as who goes to refill the water bottles in the next round.

9. Look into a personal trainer. If you have personal trainers in your area, they are skilled in keeping workouts healthy and fun. They will be in charge of designing your workout routine. All you have to do is show up! The added bonus is they get to watch the clock, which means you can devote 100 percent of yourself to simply

getting through the workout and heading home.

10.	You're allowed to reward yourself. Did you complete a full week of workouts? Rent that movie you've been wanting to see. Two weeks? It might be time for a new pair of shoes! Keep yourself motivated by setting goals and rewards- just don't reward yourself for goals not met or you'll lose your motivation.

# Chapter 6: Dealing with the Keto Flu & Other Side Effects

The keto diet proved to be a little more difficult than Elena expected. Transitioning into Ketosis was not as effortless as Janet had made it seem. In fact, Elena began to feel like she might be getting sick. She made an appointment to see her doctor, fearing she had contracted the flu.

As it turns out, Elena did have the flu- but not influenza. Elena had a set of side effects of ketosis often described as the "keto flu." It is not an uncommon threshold that dieters find themselves in when transitioning into ketosis.

Because the body is learning how to burn ketones instead of carbs, it often will go through a period of confusion. This is the body's way of telling you that it thinks it's starving. In time, though, it will balance itself out, and you'll be feeling better than ever.

Elena's doctor outlined for her the following side effects and ways to help curb them. She assured her the side effects would not last and encouraged her to stick to her diet and routine because she would soon make it through to the other side!

## Hypoglycemia:

During the period where your body is adjusting to ketosis, you might experience temporary hypoglycemia. This is because your body isn't sure how to start burning fat for energy and is instead fooled into believing you are running low on fuel.

It is not uncommon to feel brain fog, dizziness, hunger, irritability, mood swings, and fatigue. Eat smaller meals spread throughout the day during these days to keep your body feeling satisfied and don't feel bad if you have to take a nap.
You might also experience a runny nose, headaches, diarrhea, or nausea because your body could even be tricked into thinking it is fighting an illness. It's okay to take over the counter medication to help control these symptoms.

One thing you should not do, though, is give into sugar cravings. Instead, if you feel the need to eat something sweet, drink a tall glass of water. Some even chew sugar-free gum. Just don't let your body take in any bonus carbs, because that's when you will have to begin the entire process over again.

You can also try taking magnesium supplements. Magnesium helps the brain feel calmer throughout the day.

**Muscle Weakness:**

Your body is learning to use a completely new kind of fuel, so it is to be expected that it won't want to function at its top shape from the beginning. Your muscles are full of mitochondria that work to produce energy and will suddenly have to figure out how to change what they do.

It's okay to skip a workout or two until these symptoms subside. The good news is that, once they do, you'll feel stronger than ever before.

**Difficulty Sleeping:**

Because your body is adjusting, your cortisol and melatonin levels will fluctuate. These are the body's chemicals that are used to help you sleep. This might lead to bouts of insomnia in the early weeks of the keto diet. It's okay to take an over the counter sleep aid if needed, but don't let yourself become reliant on them.

## Heart Palpitations:

Again, you can blame cortisol. When cortisol spikes higher than usual, we might find our heart palpitating more than usual. Don't be frightened. Take a seat, sip a glass of cold water, and rest.

## Mineral Deficiency:

As your diet changes and your body adjusts, you might find that you are not storing all the nutrients you need. It's a good idea to purchase a daily vitamin supplement that you can include in your morning routine.

## Frequent Urination:

Not only are you drinking more water, but your body is breaking down fats, and your kidneys are changing. It would be foolish to believe that your urine won't change, as well. You will find yourself having to go more often. Plan for frequent bathroom breaks and don't try to hold it for too long. This, too, will pass.

## Constipation:

You might find that you are having more difficulty performing a different bathroom function. Work in a fiber supplement and remember not to skip out on the water, no matter how often it has you running to relieve your bladder.

## Keto Breath:

Acetone levels will spike as you are entering ketosis. They are often released in our breath, which is an unpleasant side effect. Again, this is a good time to reach for sugar-free gum. Hang in there, this symptom usually subsides by the end of the second week.

## Feelings of Hopelessness:

You might find yourself feeling like dieting isn't going to work or that you should just give up. This is actually a chemical reaction to ketosis. Don't give into it. To help Elena make it through this part of the transition, her physician gave her a print out of inspirational quotes that would remind her to stay on track to a healthier future.

# Motivational Quotes to Get You Through:

"When you think about quitting, think about why you started." -Anonymous

"Your body can stand up to almost anything. It's your mind that you have to convince."  - Anonymous

"Respect your body. It's the only one you get."- Anonymous

"Either you run the day, or the day runs you." – Jim Rohn

"Never give up, everyone has bad days. Pick yourself up and keep going."- Anonymous

"I may not be the strongest, I may not be the fastest, but I'll be darned if I'm not trying my hardest."- Anonymous

"Run when you can, walk when you have to, crawl if you must, just never give up." – Dean Karnazes

"Success belongs only to those who are willing to work harder than anyone else." – Anonymous

"Small changes can make a big difference." –
Anonymous

"Exercise is like an addiction. Once you're in it, you feel like your body needs it." – Elsa Patak

"Strive for progress, not perfection."-
Anonymous

"Don't stop when it hurts, stop when you're done."- Anonymous

"Don't wait. The time will never be just right." – Napoleon Hill

"Champions aren't made in gyms. Champions are made from something they have deep inside them – a desire, a dream, vision."- Anonymous

"Infuse your life with action. Don't wait for it to happen. Make it happen. Make your own future. Make your own hope. Make your own love. And whatever your beliefs, honor your creator, not by passively waiting for grace to come down from upon high, but by doing what you can to make grace happen... yourself, right now, right down here on Earth." -Bradley Whitford

"Accept the challenges so that you can feel the exhilaration of victory." -George S. Patton

"Action is a great restorer and builder of confidence. Inaction is not only the result but the cause, of fear. Perhaps the action you take will be successful; perhaps different action or adjustments will have to follow. But any action is better than no action at all." -Norman Vincent Peale

"Our greatest weakness lies in giving up. The most certain way to success is always to try one more time." -Thomas Edison

"Only I can change my life. No one can do it for me." -Carol Burnett

"Failure will never overtake me if my determination to succeed is strong enough." - Og Mandino

"With the new day comes new strengths and new thoughts." -Eleanor Roosevelt

"Good, better, best. Never rest. Not 'til your good is better and your better is best." -St. Jerome

"It does not matter how slowly you go as long as you do not stop." -Confucius

"You can't cross the sea merely by standing and staring at the water." -Rabindranath Tagore

"It always seems impossible until it's done." -Nelson Mandela

"Either I will find a way, or I will make one." -Philip Sidney

"Setting goals is the first step to turning the invisible into the visible." -Tony Robbins

"Problems are not stop signs. They are guidelines." -Robert H. Schuller

"We may encounter many defeats, but we must not be defeated." -Maya Angelou

"Set your goals high and don't stop 'til you get there." -Bo Jackson

"Keep your eyes on the sky and your feet on the ground." – Theodore Roosevelt

"When something is important enough, you do it even if the odds are not in your favor." -Elon Musk

"Do the difficult things while they are easy and do the great things while they are small. A journey of a thousand miles begins with just a single step." -Lao Tzu

"The most effective way to do it is just to do it." -Amelia Earhart

"Be kind to yourself whenever it is possible. It is always possible." -The Dalai Lama

"We should not give up, and we should not allow the problem to defeat us." -A. P. J. Abdul Kalam

"Never, never, never give up." -Winston Churchill

"If you fell down yesterday, stand back up today." -H. G. Wells

"Perseverance is not a long race. It is many short races, one right after the other." -Walter Elliot

"Well done is better than well said." -Benjamin Franklin

"Don't watch the clock. Do what it does. Keep moving." -Sam Levenson

"What you do today can improve all your tomorrows." -Ralph Marston

"There is only one corner of the universe that you can be certain of your ability to improve, and that is your own self." -Aldous Huxley

"By failing to prepare, you are preparing to fail." -Benjamin Franklin

"Start where you are. Do what you can. Use what you have." -Arthur Ashe

"The way to get started is to quit talking and begin doing." -Walt Disney

"Never give up, for that is just the place and time that the tide will turn." -Harriet Beecher Stowe

"Perseverance is failing 19 times and succeeding the 20th." -Julie Andrews

"The ultimate aim of the ego is not to see something, but to see something." -Muhammad Igbal

"A goal is a dream with a deadline." -Napoleon Hill

"If you don't like how things are, you can always change it! Lucky us! We are not trees!" – Jim Rohn

"You simply have to put one foot in front of the other and keep going. Put blinders on and plow right ahead." – George Lucas

"You just can't beat the person who never gives up." -Babe Ruth

"A good plan violently executed now is better than a perfect plan executed in a week." -George S. Patton

## The Broken Barrier:

Before long, Elena was feeling in better shape than ever before. By following her doctor's recommendations and turning to her inspirational quote list when needed, Catherin made it through her period of keto flu and soon felt ready to take on the world with her new, healthier future!

# Chapter 7:
# A Lifestyle Change for Elena

By summer, Elena was feeling and looking better than she had in years!

Not only had she made it back to her pre-move weight, she felt energized and ready to celebrate with her friends and family. Her Maid of Honor dress fit like a glove, and she felt attractive and radiant for the onslaught of photography on the day of the wedding.

Amidst declarations of "You look great!" Elena found time to share her keto diet experience with relatives and friends who were also in need of improving their lifestyle.

Still, Elena knew that the keto diet, alone, was not a lifelong solution.

Ketosis is not meant to last forever. In fact, it is unhealthy to maintain long-term. Your body simply cannot function for life on ketones alone and will, eventually, begin to suffer if you don't reintroduce a healthy portion of carbs into your daily life.

When Elena returned from the wedding, she knew it was time to develop a new, longer-term plan for healthier living. Slowly, she began to re-introduce carbs into her diet. She started by upping her daily carb intake slightly.

Instead of limiting herself to 35 total carbs per day, Elena began allowing herself fifty. Then, after a couple weeks of upping her carb intake from 35 to 50, she started letting herself carb-load on weekends.

On Saturdays and Sundays, Elena would allow herself 100 carbs at first. After a few weeks of adjustment, she let Saturdays and Sundays swell up to 200 carbs, but maintained her weekly carb intake at 50.

Elena was also careful to monitor the types of carbs she was eating. High glycemic carbs increase the body's insulin level. She continued to avoid sugary beverages and candy. Instead, she treated her sweet tooth with flavored oatmeal, whole grain bread with jelly, and fresh fruits. She was happy to reintroduce pasta into her diet and be able to increase the amount of fresh fruit she could consume in a day.

Once a week, Elena treated herself to a special dessert of ice cream or her favorite pastry. This kept her from feeling like she would be deprived of life and gave her something to look forward to at the end of the week. She treated this indulgence as a reward for maintaining a healthy diet and workout routine throughout the week. She knew this would prevent a junk food binge in a moment of weakness.

Elena also chose to maintain her workout routine as was already scheduled. Sometimes, she would even increase the amount of times she spent on her workouts when her schedule allowed. After getting used to her workout routine, Elena found that she looked forward to it as a regular part of her day and actually began to enjoy the way she felt post workout.

Elena timed her carb intake so that she was taking in the bulk of her carbs in her post workout meals. This meant that her carbs were being burned instead of stored. She opted to continue to eat low or zero carb meals at dinner to avoid "sleeping with the enemy."

As Elena introduced carbs into her diet, she remembered one crucial piece of advice that many keto dieters forget. Inevitably, forgetting this step leads to rapid weight gain back. Elena, under the advice of Janet and her physician, knew that as carbs were reintroduced, she would need to lower her daily fat intake.

The calorie hike when carbs are reintroduced is nothing to scoff at! Don't cut fats completely, but limit them to a healthy portion and be mindful of saturated fats. Elena found success in staggering her meals. She alternated between healthy fat and protein and low-glycemic carbs and protein. In doing so, her body was able to readjust effortlessly.

It goes without saying that what works for Elena may or may not work for everyone, including yourself. Elena's story should simply be used as a guideline by which you can form your own plan.

Be sure to consult your physician, stick to your plan, and your success is guaranteed!

# Meal Plan & Grocery List:

If you are feeling overwhelmed by all of the information, feel free to borrow your first two weeks of keto dieting from Elena. The meal plan and grocery list are enclosed for your convenience. You can feel confident borrowing all or any part of the plan as it suits your needs.

## Meal Plan

Below, you will find the meal plan Elena used to begin her Keto diet. Elena started on a Sunday, but you can start any day of the week. Feel free to switch the days as you see fit to maximize efficiency for your busy schedule!

| Day 1 | |
|---|---|
| Breakfast | Sunday Breakfast Platter |
| AM Snack | Sugar-Free Gelatin |
| Lunch | Italian Leftwich |
| PM Snack | Jerky |
| Dinner | Eggplant Rollatini |

|  Day 2 | |
| --- | --- |
| Breakfast | Probiotic Berry Smoothie |
| AM Snack | ½ Avocado |
| Lunch | Cream Cheese Pinwheels |
| PM Snack | Pickle |
| Dinner | Chicken Avocado Casserole |

|  Day 3 | |
| --- | --- |
| Breakfast | Vanilla Mint Smoothie |
| AM Snack | String Cheese |
| Lunch | Avocado Egg Salad |
| PM Snack | Pork Rinds |
| Dinner | Chicken in White Sauce |

|  Day 4 | |
| --- | --- |
| Breakfast | Spinach & Grape Smoothie |
| AM Snack | Cocoa Nibs |
| Lunch | Garlic Pancetta Chicken Salad |
| PM Snack | Walnuts |
| Dinner | Keto Reuben Skillet |

|  Day 5 | |
| --- | --- |
| Breakfast | Probiotic Berry Smoothie |
| AM Snack | Cocoa Nibs |
| Lunch | Italian Keto Platter |
| PM Snack | Pork Rinds |
| Dinner | Philly Cheesesteak Wrap |

| Day 6 | |
|---|---|
| Breakfast | Vanilla Mint Smoothie |
| AM Snack | Sugar-Free Gelatin |
| Lunch | Keto-Friendly Roast Beef Sandwich |
| PM Snack | Walnuts |
| Dinner | Crockpot Chicken Stew |

| Day 7 | |
|---|---|
| Breakfast | Saturday Breakfast Platter |
| AM Snack | String Cheese |
| Lunch | Roast Beef and Cheddar Platter |
| PM Snack | ½ Avocado |
| Dinner | Southwestern Shephard's Pie |

| Day 8 | |
|---|---|
| Breakfast | Sunday Breakfast Platter |
| AM Snack | ½ Avocado |
| Lunch | Sriracha Broccoli Salad |
| PM Snack | Pork Rinds |
| Dinner | Beef Satay |

| Day 9 | |
|---|---|
| Breakfast | Spinach & Grape Smoothie |
| AM Snack | Cocoa Nibs |
| Lunch | Avocado Tuna Salad |
| PM Snack | Pickle |
| Dinner | Ribeye Steak Salad |

| Day 10 | |
| --- | --- |
| Breakfast | Probiotic Berry Smoothie |
| AM Snack | Sugar-Free Gelatin |
| Lunch | Coleslaw Wraps |
| PM Snack | ½ Avocado |
| Dinner | Mini Chicken Pot Pies |

| Day 11 | |
| --- | --- |
| Breakfast | Vanilla Mint Smoothie |
| AM Snack | ½ Avocado |
| Lunch | Chicken & Cabbage Plate |
| PM Snack | Jerky |
| Dinner | Stuffed Peppers |

| Day 12 | |
| --- | --- |
| Breakfast | Spinach & Grape Smoothie |
| AM Snack | Cocoa Nibs |
| Lunch | Chicken Salad Stuffed Eggs |
| PM Snack | Pork Rinds |
| Dinner | BLT Salad |

| Day 13 | |
| --- | --- |
| Breakfast | Probiotic Berry Smoothie |
| AM Snack | String Cheese |
| Lunch | Bright Stir Fry |
| PM Snack | Walnuts |
| Dinner | Keto Friendly Sliders |

| Day 14 | |
|---|---|
| Breakfast | Saturday Breakfast Platter |
| AM Snack | ½ Avocado |
| Lunch | Magic 5 Keto Salad |
| PM Snack | ½ Avocado |
| Dinner | Sausage & Cabbage Melt |

** Remember, several of these meals will be made much easier by cooking and shredding the chicken ahead of time. Put the chicken breasts in the crockpot and cook them for several hours. Cool, shred with a fork, and separate into one-cup bags. You'll thank yourself later!

# Grocery List

Below, you will find the organized shopping list for all the ingredients Elena used on her two-week diet plan. Before you become overwhelmed by the size of the list, remember a few key things:

1. **Most of this is already in your kitchen.**
   Go take a look. This is a list of all the things you will need, but it doesn't necessarily have to be a list of things you purchase. If you already have it, cross it off and don't worry!

2. **There will be extra for next time.**
   It's impossible to buy ingredients in the exact quantities you want. Everything on this list is rounded up to ensure you have what you need, but that also means you won't have to buy as much on your next trip.

3. **Look for sales!**
   In- season produce is always a good buy. Meat sales typically run in the mornings. Remember the hints Elena researched and listed earlier and this shopping trip will be a breeze.

Without further ado, enjoy your shopping trip!

Dairy/Cooler
3 Dozen Eggs
5 Cups Coconut Milk
5 Cups Almond Milk
1 Bag String Cheese
2.5 lbs Provolone Cheese
16 oz. Cream Cheese
American Cheese Singles
3.5 lbs. Cheddar Cheese
2.5 lbs. Mozzarella
1 lb. Butter
4 Small Cartons Heavy Cream
½ lb. Colby Jack Cheese
1 Container Grated Parmesan Cheese
8 oz. Sour Cream
4 oz. Feta Cheese
Small Container Cottage Cheese

Pantry
Coffee
4 cups Kombucha Tea
Vanilla Extract
4 oz. Pork Rinds
1 lb. Cocoa Nibs
½ lb. Walnuts
1 Jar Dill Pickles, Whole
Six Pack Sugar-Free Gelatin Cups

1 Large Jar of Mayonnaise
1 Bottle of Olive Oil
1 Bottle of Mustard
3 Small Cans Tuna in Oil
1 Jar Pepperoncini Peppers
1 Bottle of Dijon Mustard
1 Jar Pickle Relish
Coconut Oil
Soy Sauce
Apple Cider Vinegar
1 Small Bag Dry Roasted Sunflower Seeds
Sriracha Sauce
2 Cartons Chicken Stock
White Wine Vinegar
Coconut Flour
Almond Flour
Baking Powder
Worchestire Sauce
1 Jar Jalapeno Peppers
Chili Sauce
1 Can Tomato Sauce
Small Bottle Honey
1 Jar Smooth Peanut Butter
1 Can Sauerkraut

Meat
3 lbs. Bacon
Small Bag Unflavored Beef Jerky
14 Chicken Breasts (to cook in crockpot ahead
of time)

4 Chicken Breasts to prepare whole later
2 lbs. Roast Beef Deli Meat
1 lb. Thin-Sliced Salami
¼ lb. Deli Sliced Turkey
¼ lb. Deli Sliced Ham
6 oz. Ham Steak
¼ lb. Pepperoni
8 oz. Prosciutto
1 lb. Ground Turkey
2 lbs. Ground Sausage
8 oz. Ribeye Steak
2.5 lbs. Ground Beef
1 lb. Flank Steak
1 lb. Deli- Sliced Corned Beef


<u>Spices</u>
Salt
Cumin
Pepper
Cilantro
Lemon Pepper
Thyme
Steak Seasoning
Paprika
Coriander
Curry
Red Pepper Flakes
Parsley
Basil

<u>Produce</u>
3 Cups Grapes
12 Cups Baby Spinach
21 Avocados
4 Cups Blueberries
4 Cups Cherries
1 Cup Fresh Mint
3 Limes
2 Cups Mushrooms
2 Heads Red Cabbage
2 Large Eggplants
8 Red Onions
3 Heads of Lettuce
1 Container Guacamole
1 Cucumber
6 oz. Fresh Cilantro
3 Lemons
6 Cloves Garlic
1 lb. Carrots
3 Red Bell Peppers
4 Green Bell Peppers
2 lbs. Fresh Green Beans
1 lb. Collard Leaves
1 lb. Alfalfa Sprouts
4 Cups Spring Mix
4 Heads Broccoli
8 Radishes
1 Bundle Scallions
2 Tomatoes
1 Bundle Celery

1 lb. Fresh Peas
1 Head Green Cabbage
2 Cups Green Salad Mix
1 Head Cauliflower

<u>Extras</u>
Toothpicks
Bamboo Skewers

# Breakfast Recipes & Snacks

## Sunday Morning Breakfast Platter

This recipe needs 10 minutes to prepare, 10 minutes to cook and will make 1 serving.

- Protein: 50 grams
- Net Carbs: 10 grams
- Fats: 30 grams

*What to Use*

- Eggs (2 large)
- Ham Steak (3 oz.)
- Black Coffee (1 cup)
- Stevia Sweetener (to taste)
- Salt and Pepper (to taste)

*What to Do*

- In a hot frying pan, cook your ham steak until browned on each side.
- In the same frying pan, cook your eggs over easy using the grease left from the ham.
- Salt and pepper your platter and sweeten your coffee as desired.

# Probiotic Berry Smoothie

This recipe needs 15 minutes to prepare, 0 minutes to cook and will make 4 servings. Extra servings may be frozen in freezer bags, then thawed and consumed at a later date.

- Protein: 3 grams
- Net Carbs: 9 grams
- Fats: 17 grams

*What to Use*

- Fresh Baby Spinach (1 cup)
- Kombucha Tea (1 cup)
- Coconut Milk (1/2 cup)
- Avocado (1 fruit)
- Blueberries (1 cup)
- Cherries (1 cup)

*What to Do*

- Place all ingredients in a blender and liquify to desired consistency.
- Separate into four servings.
- Freeze the extra in individual freezer bags to be used later.

# Vanilla Mint Smoothie

This recipe needs 15 minutes to prepare, 0 minutes to cook and will make 4 servings. Extra servings may be frozen in freezer bags, then thawed and consumed at a later date.

- Protein: 3 grams
- Net Carbs: 8 grams
- Fats: 25 grams

*What to Use*

- Avocado (1 fruit)
- Coconut Milk (1 cup)
- Almond Milk (1 cup)
- Stevia Sweetener (1 tablespoon)
- Fresh Mint (1/4 cup, chopped)
- Cilantro (1 tablespoon)
- Lime Juice (1 fruit)
- Ice (4 cubes)
- Vanilla Extract (1 tablespoon)

*What to Do*

- Place all ingredients in a blender and liquify to desired consistency.
- Separate into four servings.

- Freeze the extra in individual freezer bags
  to be used later.

# Spinach & Grape Smoothie

This recipe needs 15 minutes to prepare, 0 minutes to cook and will make 4 servings. Extra servings may be frozen in freezer bags, then thawed and consumed at a later date.

- Protein: 16 grams
- Net Carbs: 6 grams
- Fats: 22 grams

*What to Use*

- Eggs (2 large)
- Almond Milk (1/2 cup)
- Grapes (1 cup)
- Fresh Spinach (1 cup)
- Avocado (1 fruit)
- Ice (8 cubes)

*What to Do*

- Place all ingredients in a blender and liquify to desired consistency.
- Separate into four servings.
- Freeze the extra in individual freezer bags to be used later.

# Saturday Morning Breakfast Platter

This recipe needs 15 minutes to prepare, 30 minutes to cook and will make 6 servings.
- Protein: 21 grams
- Net Carbs: 2 grams
- Fats: 20 grams

*What to Use*
- Egg (1 large)
- Bacon (2 strips)
- Mushrooms (1/2 cup)
- Black Coffee (1 cup)
- Stevia Sweetener (to taste)
- Salt and Pepper (to taste)

*What to Do*
- In a hot frying pan, cook your bacon until crisp.
- In the same frying pan, scramble your egg and sauté your mushrooms in bacon grease
- Salt and pepper your platter and sweeten your coffee as desired.

# Zero Prep Snack List

- 1 oz. Pork Rinds (0 carbs, 9 g. protein, 5 g. fat)
- String Cheese (1 carbs, 8 g. protein, 6 g. fat)
- 1 oz. Jerky- no added flavor (4 carbs, 12 g. protein, 1 g. fat)
- ½ cup Cocoa Nibs (4 carbs, 3 g. protein, 6 g. fat)
- 1 oz. Walnuts (2.8 carbs, 7 g. protein, 17 g. fat)
- ½ Avocado with salt & pepper (7 carbs, 1 g. protein, 20 g. fat)
- 1 Whole Dill Pickle (2 carbs, 0 g. protein, 0 g. fat)
- Sugar-Free Jell-O Quick Cup (0 carbs, 1 g. protein, 0 g. fat)

# Lunch Recipes

## Chicken and Cabbage Plate

This recipe needs 5 minutes to prepare, 0 minutes to cook and will make 2 servings.

- Protein: 48 grams
- Net Carbs: 7 grams
- Fats: 91 grams

*What to Use*

- Fresh Red Cabbage (7 oz.)
- Red Onion (1/2 medium size)
- Chicken Breasts (1 cup, cooked and shredded)
- Mayonnaise (1/2 cup)
- Olive Oil (1 tablespoon)
- Salt and Pepper (to taste)

*What to Do*

- Shred the cabbage and arrange on the plate as a bottom layer to your salad.
- Slice the onion and add it as the second layer with the shredded rotisserie chicken.
- Add a dollop of mayonnaise to the top.

- Drizzle olive oil over the cabbage and add salt and pepper to taste.

# Keto-Friendly Roast Beef Sandwich

This recipe needs 5 minutes to prepare, 0 minutes to cook and will make 1 serving.

- Protein: 41 grams
- Net Carbs: 2 grams
- Fats: 14 grams

*What to Use*

- Roast Beef Deli Meat (4 oz.)
- Mustard (1 tablespoon)
- Lettuce (1 large leaf)
- Provolone Cheese (1 slice)

*What to Do*

- Lay out the large lettuce leaf.
- Spread mustard over the leaf.
- Add the roast beef and slice of gouda cheese.
- Roll the lettuce leaf around the inner ingredients.

# Avocado Egg Salad

This recipe needs 5 minutes to prepare, 10 minutes to cook and will make 1 serving.

- Protein: 7 grams
- Net Carbs: 5 grams
- Fats: 14 grams

*What to Use*

- Egg (1 large)
- Mayonnaise (1 teaspoon)
- Guacamole (2 tablespoons)
- Salt and Pepper (to taste)

*What to Do*

- Hard boil your egg.
- Dice egg into a bowl.
- Add guacamole, mayonnaise, and salt and pepper.
- Mix ingredients together and enjoy.

# Cream Cheese Pinwheels

This recipe needs 10 minutes to prepare, 00 minutes to cook and will make 3 servings.

- Protein: 8 grams
- Net Carbs: 2 grams
- Fats: 12 grams

*What to Use*

- Cream Cheese (8 oz. block)
- Pickle Relish (4 tablespoons)
- Thin Sliced Salami (8-10 slices)

*What to Do*

- Bring cream cheese to room temperature and then whip to a fluffy consistency.
- Spread the cream cheese ¼ inch thick on a piece of plastic wrap.
- Spread pickle relish over the cream cheese.
- Place the salami over the cream cheese and relish, overlapping the slices, so the cream cheese is completely covered.
- Place a second piece of plastic wrap over the salami and press down until all ingredients are sealed together inside.
- Flip the entire rectangle over so the cream cheese is now face up.

- Carefully peel back the plastic wrap and begin rolling all ingredients into a log. Make sure you are removing all plastic wrap as you go.
- Place pinwheel in a tight plastic wrap roll and refrigerate overnight.
- Slice the log into pinwheels of your preferred thickness.

# Italian Leftwich

This recipe needs 15 minutes to prepare, 00 minutes to cook and will make 1 serving.

- Protein: 21 grams
- Net Carbs: 4 grams
- Fats: 17 grams

*What to Use*

- Lettuce leaf (1 large)
- American Cheese (1 slice)
- Deli- Sliced Turkey (3 slices)
- Deli- Sliced Ham (3 slices)
- Pepperoni (4 Slices)
- Pepperoncini Pepper (1, chopped)

*What to Do*

- Stack ingredients on top of lettuce leaf and roll them together with the leaf on the outside.

# Avocado Tuna Salad

This recipe needs 10 minutes to prepare, 00 minutes to cook and will make 6 servings.

- Protein: 21 grams
- Net Carbs: 8 grams
- Fats: 24 grams

*What to Use*

- Tuna in Oil (3 small cans)
- Cucumber (1 sliced)
- Avocados (2, peeled and sliced)
- Cilantro (1/4 cup, chopped)
- Lemon Juice (2 tablespoons)
- Red Onion (1, thinly sliced)
- Olive Oil (2 tablespoons)
- Salt and Pepper (to taste)

*What to Do*

- Combine cucumber, avocado, tuna, cilantro, and red onion in a large bowl.
- Drizzle with lemon juice, olive oil, salt, and pepper.
- Toss to combinc thc ingredients.

# Roast Beef & Cheddar Platter

This recipe needs 5 minutes to prepare, 0 minutes to cook and will make 2 servings.

- Protein: 38 grams
- Net Carbs: 6 grams
- Fats: 98 grams

*What to Use*

- Radishes (6)
- Avocado (1)
- Scallion (1)
- Cheddar Cheese (5 oz)
- Deli-Sliced Roast Beef (7 oz)
- Lettuce (2 oz.)
- Dijon Mustard (1 tablespoon)
- Mayonnaise (1/2 cup)
- Olive Oil (2 tablespoons)
- Salt and Pepper (to taste)

*What to Do*

- Place cheese, meat, avocado, and radishes on a plate.
- Pile on mayonnaise, mustard, and onion.
- Drizzle with olive oil.
- Serve with lettuce leaves for wrapping.

# Chicken Salad Stuffed Eggs

This recipe needs 10 minutes to prepare, 10 minutes to cook and will make 2 servings.

- Protein: 34 grams
- Net Carbs: 5 grams
- Fats: 20 grams

*What to Use*

- Eggs (6)
- Shredded leftover Chicken (1 cup)
- Mayonnaise (2 tablespoons)
- Minced Onion (1 tablespoon)
- Dijon Mustard (1 teaspoon)
- Pickle Relish (2 tablespoons)
- Lemon Pepper (to taste)

*What to Do*

- Boil, peel, and split your eggs.
- Scoop out yolks and toss them away.
- In a large bowl, combine all other ingredients except lemon pepper.
- Refrigerate chicken salad mixture until cooled.
- Scoop chicken salad into egg white halves in the same way you would for deviled eggs.

- Sprinkle with lemon pepper to taste.

# Italian Keto Platter

This recipe needs 5 minutes to prepare, 0 minutes to cook and will make 2 servings.

- Protein: 40 grams
- Net Carbs: 6 grams
- Fats: 70 grams
- Calories: 275

*What to Use*

- Green Olives (8)
- Olive Oil (1/3 cup)
- Tomato (1, thinly sliced)
- Prosciutto (8 oz., thinly sliced)
- Mozzarella Cheese (8 oz.)
- Salt and Pepper (to taste)

*What to Do*

- Pot prosciutto, cheese, tomatoes, and olives on a plate.
- Drizzle with olive oil and season with salt and pepper to taste.

# Bright Stir Fry

This recipe needs 10 minutes to prepare, 15 minutes to cook and will make 4 servings.

- Protein: 12 grams
- Net Carbs: 8 grams
- Fats: 15 grams

*What to Use*

- Coconut oil (1/4 cup)
- Garlic (2 cloves, minced)
- Carrots (2, peeled and thinly sliced)
- Radishes (2, thinly sliced)
- Red Bell Pepper (2, thinly sliced)
- Fresh Green Beans (2 cups)
- Shredded leftover chicken (2 cups)
- Salt & Pepper (to taste)
- Soy Sauce (to taste, but no more than 2 tablespoons)

*What to Do*

- Sauté onion in coconut oil for five minutes.
- Add the garlic and cook over medium heat for 1 minute.

- Add carrots, peppers, radishes, and green beans and cook over medium until vegetables cook through.
- Add soy sauce, salt, and pepper to taste.

# Coleslaw Wraps

This recipe needs 30 minutes to prepare, 00 minutes to cook and will make 4 servings.

- Protein: 37 grams
- Net Carbs: 7 grams
- Fats: 22 grams

*What to Use for Coleslaw*

- Red Cabbage (3 cups, thinly sliced)
- Diced Scallions (1/2 cup)
- Mayonnaise (3/4 cup)
- Apple Cider Vinegar (2 teaspoons)
- Salt and Pepper (to taste)

*What to Use for Wraps & Filling*

- Collard Leaves (16, steamed)
- Alfalfa Sprouts (1/2 cup)
- Ground Turkey (1 lb., cooked and chilled)
- Toothpicks (for holding wraps together)

*What to Do*

- Combine coleslaw ingredients well and chill.
- Remove stems from collard greens. This will leave a split halfway through the leaf. That's okay.
- Place a spoonful of coleslaw on the full half of the leaf, then a spoonful of meat and top with sprouts.
- Tuck the sides of the split half of the leaf and then roll to keep the filling from spilling out.
- Insert a toothpick into the roll to keep it together.
- Refrigerate for at least ½ hour.

# Magic 5 Keto Salad

This recipe needs 10 minutes to prepare, 10 minutes to cook and will make 2 servings.

- Protein: 39 grams
- Net Carbs: 8 grams
- Fats: 44 grams

*What to Use*

- Bacon (3 strips)
- Avocado (1 fruit)
- Spring Mix (4 cups)
- Chicken Breasts (2 cups, cooked and shredded)
- Olive Oil (2 tablespoons)
- Apple Cider Vinegar (2 tablespoons)
- Salt and Pepper (to taste)

*What to Do*

- Mix apple cider, salt, and pepper together in a bowl.
- Cook bacon, adding ½ bacon grease to Apple Cider, salt, and pepper mixture.
- Pile Spring Mix, Chicken, Bacon (crumbled) and Avocado in a separate bowl.
- Drizzle with the liquid mixture.

## Sriracha Broccoli Salad

This recipe needs 15 minutes to prepare, 0 minutes to cook and will make 4 servings.

- Protein: 10 grams
- Net Carbs: 6 grams
- Fats: 16 grams

*What to Use*

- Broccoli (4 cups, chopped)
- Mayonnaise (1 cup)
- Red Bell Pepper (1/2, sliced and cored)
- Cheddar Cheese (1/4 cup, shredded)
- Bacon (6 slices, baked and crumbled)
- Dry Roasted Sunflower Seeds (1/4 cup)
- Apple Cider Vinegar (1/2 teaspoon)
- Sriracha Sauce (1/2 tablespoon)
- Salt and Pepper to taste

*What to Do*

- Toss all ingredients together in a large bowl.
- Store in sealed container in the refrigerator for at least two hours.

# Garlic Pancetta Chicken Salad

This recipe needs 15 minutes to prepare, 0 minutes to cook and will make 4 servings.

- Protein: 35 grams
- Net Carbs: 1 gram
- Fats: 46 grams

*What to Use*

- Chicken Breasts (2 cups, cooked and shredded)
- Olive Oil (1 tablespoon)
- Lettuce (4 large leaves)
- Minced Garlic (2 cloves)
- Provolone Cheese (3 oz, shredded or grated)
- Salt and Pepper to taste

*What to Do*

- Lay lettuce leaves out flat.
- Combine chicken breasts, olive oil, minced garlic, cheese, salt and pepper in a bowl.
- Spread inside lettuce leaves and roll into wraps.

# Dinner Recipes

## Stuffed Peppers

This recipe needs 15 minutes to prepare, 45 minutes to cook and will make 2 servings.

- Protein: 35 grams
- Net Carbs: 11 grams
- Fats: 30 grams

*What to Use*

- Green Bell Peppers (2, cored but not sliced)
- Onion (1 small)
- Ground Sausage (1/2 pound)
- Cheddar Cheese (1.5 oz, shredded)
- Cream Cheese (2 oz.)
- Eggs (2)

*What to Do*

- Stand your bell peppers up on parchment paper on a baking sheet, cored but unsliced to create bowls.

- Cook your ground sausage and onion together in a skillet until sausage is fully cooked and onion becomes clear.
- Layer 1 oz. cream cheese in the bottom of each bell pepper.
- Scoop half of your meat mixture into each bell pepper on top of the cream cheese layer.
- Layer the top with shredded cheddar cheese.
- Bake the peppers for 20 minutes at 375 degrees.
- Break open one egg into the top of each pepper. Return to oven and bake an additional ten minutes.

# Mini Chicken Pot Pies

This recipe needs 45 minutes to prepare, 30 minutes to cook and will make 12 servings.
- Protein: 23 grams
- Net Carbs: 61 grams
- Fats: 36 grams

*What to Use for Filling*
- Chicken Breasts (2 cups, cooked and shredded)
- Butter (2 tablespoons)
- Celery (2 stalks, finely chopped)
- Onion (1 medium, diced)
- Carrot (1/2 cup, coarsely grated)
- Dried Thyme (1/4 teaspoon)
- Chicken Stock (1/2 cup)
- White Wine Vinegar (1 tablespoon)
- Heavy Cream (1 ½ cup)
- Fresh Peas (1/2 cup)
- Paprika (2 teaspoons)
- Salt and Pepper to taste

*What to Use for Crust*
- Coconut flour (1/2 cup)

- Almond flour (1/2 cup)
- Baking Powder (2 teaspoons)
- Salt (1/4 teaspoon)
- Dried Thyme (1/4 teaspoon)
- Eggs (2 large)
- Mozzarella Cheese (3 cups, grated)
- Butter (10 tablespoons)

*What to Do*

- For filling, combine chicken breasts, butter, dried thyme, chicken stock, paprika, salt, and pepper in a bowl.
- For filling, heat all other ingredients over the stove until boiling and cooked through, then mix into bowl ingredients. Let cool.
- For crusts, mix flours, salt, thyme, eggs, and butter in a bowl. This will create a flaky dough.
- Press dough into greased muffin tins, creating cups.
- Fill cups with filling, top with mozzarella cheese, and bake 30 minutes at 350 degrees.

# Sausage and Cabbage Melt

This recipe needs 15 minutes to prepare, 40 minutes to cook and will make 4 servings.

- Protein: 18 grams
- Net Carbs: 3 grams
- Fats: 15 grams

*What to Use*

- Sausage (1 lb. ground)
- Green Cabbage (1 ½ cups, shredded)
- Red Cabbage (1 ½ cups, shredded)
- Onion (1/2 cup, diced)
- Coconut Oil (2 tablespoons)
- Colby Jack Cheese (2 oz., shredded)
- Fresh Cilantro (2 tablespoons, chopped)

*What to Do*

- In cast iron skillet, heat sausage, cabbages, onion, and coconut oil until cooked through (about 20 minutes), stirring occasionally.
- Sprinkle top with cheese and cilantro.
- Place in oven to bake for an additional 20 minutes at 350 degrees.

# Ribeye Steak Salad

This recipe needs 5 minutes to prepare, 15 minutes to cook and will make 2 servings.

- Protein: 25 grams
- Net Carbs: 2 grams
- Fats: 2 grams

*What to Use*

- Ribeye Steak (8 oz.)
- Steak Seasoning (1 tablespoon)
- Green Salad Mix (2 cups)
- Olive Oil (1 tablespoon)
- White Wine Vinegar (1 teaspoon)
- Salt and Pepper to taste

*What to Do*

- Season your steak with the seasoning.
- Cook your steak to the desired doneness.
- Slice your steak into thin slices.
- On a plate, layer your steak slices over a bed of green salad mix.
- In a bowl, combine white wine vinegar, olive oil, and salt and pepper.
- Drizzle liquid over your salad.

# Philly Cheesesteak Wrap

This recipe needs 15 minutes to prepare, 0 minutes to cook and will make 4 servings.

- Protein: 28 grams
- Net Carbs: 2 grams
- Fats: 32 grams

*What to Use*

- Lettuce (4 large leaves)
- Deli Sliced Roast Beef (8 oz.)
- Mushrooms (2 oz, cooked)
- Green Bell Pepper (1, cored and sliced)
- Onion (1 oz, thin sliced)
- Olive Oil (1 tablespoon)
- Worchestire Sauce (1 tablespoon)
- Provolone Cheese (4 oz., sliced)

*What to Do*

- Lay lettuce leaves out flat.
- Layer deli meat, mushrooms, green pepper, onion, and cheese on a lettuce wrap.
- Combine Worchestire sauce and olive oil and drizzle over ingredients.
- Wrap lettuce leaves around inner ingredients to create a wrap.

# Easy Crockpot Chicken Stew

This recipe needs 5 minutes to prepare, 120 minutes to cook and will make 4 servings.

- Protein: 23 grams
- Net Carbs: 6 grams
- Fats: 11 grams

*What to Use*

- Chicken Stock (2 cups)
- Carrots (1/2 cup, peeled and diced)
- Celery Sticks (1 cup, diced)
- Onion (1/2 cup, diced)
- Chicken Breasts (2 cups, cooked and shredded)
- Garlic (3 cloves, minced)
- Thyme (1/4 teaspoon)
- Oregano (1/2 teaspoon)
- Fresh Spinach (1 cup)
- Heavy Cream (1/2 cup)
- Salt and Pepper to taste

*What to Do*

- Place all ingredients except heavy cream and spinach in the crockpot and cook on high for two hours.

- Stir in spinach and heavy cream.
- Cook an additional thirty minutes on low.

# Southwestern Shepherd's Keto Pie

This recipe needs 30 minutes to prepare, 30 minutes to cook and will make 6 servings.
- Protein: 42 grams
- Net Carbs: 4 grams
- Fats: 21 grams

*What to Use for Base*
- Bacon (4 slices, cut into small pieces)
- Ground Beef (1 lb.)
- Green Pepper (1 whole, cored and diced)
- Jalapeno Pepper (1 whole, diced)
- Chili Sauce (1 tablespoon)
- Cumin (1 teaspoon)
- Oregano (1 teaspoon)
- Onion (1/2 cup, sliced)
- Garlic (2 cloves, minced)
- Tomato Sauce (1 cup)
- Eggs (2 large)

*What to Use for Top Layer*
- Cauliflower (10 oz., chopped)
- Chicken Broth (4 tablespoons)

- Cheddar Cheese (2 ½ oz., shredded)
- Butter (3 tablespoons)
- Parmesan Cheese (3 tablespoons, grated)
- Heavy Cream (2 tablespoons)
- Salt & Pepper to taste

*What to Do*

- In a large pan, cook bacon, beef, and onions together.
- Add eggs, scrambling them into the meat.
- Add all other ingredients, heating until boiling.
- Pour chili base into the bottom of a 9x13 baking dish and set aside.
- Boil cauliflower until tender.
- Drain cauliflower and add all other ingredients. Mix with a mixer until mashed potato is thick.
- Spread cauliflower mixture over chili base.
- Bake for 20 minutes at 325 degrees.

# Chicken Avocado Casserole

This recipe needs 15 minutes to prepare, 20 minutes to cook and will make 6 servings.

- Protein: 40 grams
- Net Carbs: 6 grams
- Fats: 39 grams

*What to Use*

- Chicken Breasts (2 cups, cooked and shredded)
- Avocados (3, peeled, pitted and chopped)
- Onion (1 medium, chopped)
- Hot Sauce (1 tablespoon)
- Red Bell Pepper (1, chopped and cored)
- Sour Cream (8 oz.)
- Cheddar Cheese (8 oz., shredded)
- Salt and Pepper to taste

*What to Do*

- Mix all ingredients except cheese together into a baking dish.
- Sprinkle cheese over the top.
- Bake at 350 degrees for 20 minutes.

# Beef Satay

This recipe needs 30 minutes to prepare, 10 minutes to cook and will make 4 servings.

- Protein: 28 grams
- Net Carbs: 4 grams
- Fats: 27 grams

*What to Use for Satay & Marinade*

- Flank Steak (1 lb.)
- Soy Sauce (2 tablespoons)
- Honey (2 tablespoons)
- Coriander (1/2 teaspoon)
- Red Pepper Flakes (2 teaspoons)
- Olive Oil (1 tablespoon)
- Bamboo Skewers soaked in water

*What to Use for Peanut Sauce*

- Smooth Peanut Butter (1/4 cup)
- Coconut Milk (1/3 cup)
- Chili Sauce (1 teaspoon)
- Honey (1 tablespoon)
- Curry (1/2 teaspoon)

*What to Do*

- Cut your flank steak into 1 ½ inch strips perpendicular to the grain of the meat.
- Push the skewers through the meat, leaving a handle.
- Mix all marinade ingredients in a bowl.
- Coat the meat in the marinade and let it sit for at least fifteen minutes.
- While the meat is marinating, warm the peanut butter in a microwave-safe bowl until soft. Stir in the chili sauce, honey, and curry.
- Slowly add coconut milk to the peanut butter mixture while stirring with a whisk.
- Pour olive oil over the beef and coat all sides.
- Place skewered meat on the grill and cook until done, flipping halfway through the cooking process.

# Eggplant Rollatini

This recipe needs 15 minutes to prepare, 45 minutes to cook and will make 8 servings.
- Protein: 24 grams
- Net Carbs: 9 grams
- Fats: 28 grams

*What to Use*
- Eggplants (2, sliced lengthwise)
- Marinara Sauce (1 cup)
- Eggs (2 large)
- Fresh Spinach (3 cups)
- Feta Cheese (4 oz)
- Oregano (1 teaspoon)
- Parsley (1 teaspoon)
- Basil (1 teaspoon)
- Parmesan Cheese (2 cups, grated)
- Cottage Cheese (1 cup)
- Salt and Pepper to taste

*What to Do*
- Preheat oven to 450 degrees.
- Place eggplant slices in a parchment-lined baking sheet and sprinkle with salt and pepper.

- Bake for 15 minutes, remove and allow to cool.
- Reduce heat to 400 degrees.
- In a bowl, mix eggs, feta cheese, spinach, oregano, basil, parsley, 1 cup parmesan, and ½ cup cottage cheese until well combined.
- Pour ½ cup marinara into a 9x13 baking sheet, coating the bottom.
- Place ¼ cheese mixture onto one side of sliced eggplant, then roll up and transfer to baking dish, setting on top of the marinara bed.
- Continue doing this until pan is full.
- Cover with remaining cheese and marinara sauce.
- Bake 25 minutes and cool for 10 before serving.

# BLT Salad

This recipe needs 5 minutes to prepare, 10 minutes to cook and will make 1 servings.

- Protein: 26 grams
- Net Carbs: 4 grams
- Fats: 26 grams

## What to Use

- Tomato (2 oz, diced into cubes)
- Spinach (1 cup)
- Mozzarella Cheese (1/2 cup, shredded)
- Bacon (3 slices)

## What to Do

- Cook bacon in a skillet until crispy. Set aside until cool and crumble.
- Cook spinach in bacon grease.
- Stir crisp bacon pieces into cooked spinach, then transfer to plate.
- Sprinkle with tomato and cheese.

# Chicken in White Sauce

This recipe needs 10 minutes to prepare, 40 minutes to cook and will make 4 servings.

- Protein: 18 grams
- Net Carbs: 6 grams
- Fats: 30 grams

*What to Use*

- Chicken Breasts (4)
- Coconut Milk (1/2 cup)
- White Wine (1 cup)
- Mushrooms (3 oz)
- Fresh Green Beans (3 oz, halved)
- Dijon Mustard (2 tablespoons)
- Garlic (4 cloves, minced)
- Olive Oil (1/4 cup)
- Thyme (1 teaspoon)
- Salt & Pepper to taste

*What to Do*

- Preheat oven to 350 degrees.
- Pour half the olive oil into a frying pan and heat over medium heat.
- Add chicken breasts and cook each side for 2 minutes.

- Place chicken in a baking tray and bake for 15 minutes.
- In the same frying pan, combine mushrooms, olive oil, and garlic.
- Add beans, coconut milk, white wine, Dijon mustard, thyme, salt and pepper and mix in the pan, then reduce to simmer. The sauce will seem watery but will reduce to a sauce.
- Once the chicken is done, plate the chicken and cover with sauce.

# Keto Reuben Skillet

This recipe needs 5 minutes to prepare, 10 minutes to cook and will make 2 servings.

- Protein: 58 grams
- Net Carbs: 3 grams
- Fats: 93 grams

*What to Use*

- Butter (2 tablespoons)
- Deli Sliced Corned Beef (2/3 lb.)
- Sauerkraut (9 oz., drained)
- Dijon Mustard (1 tablespoon)
- Mayonnaise (1/2 cup)
- Swiss Cheese (4 oz.)
- Pickle Relish (4 tablespoons)

*What to Do*

- Heat up butter in a cast iron skillet over medium heat.
- Add corned beef and fry until browned on both sides.
- Drain sauerkraut and distribute evenly in pan over meat.
- Place mustard and Swiss cheese in the pan, stirring until spread evenly.

- Remove from heat and mix in mayonnaise
  and pickle relish.

# Cheeseburger Sliders

This recipe needs 15 minutes to prepare, 15 minutes to cook and will make 4 servings.

- Protein: 22 grams
- Net Carbs: 0 grams
- Fats: 21 grams

*What to Use*

- Lettuce (4 large leaves, cut in half)
- Ground Beef (1.5 lbs.)
- Egg (1)
- Worchestire Sauce (2 tablespoons)
- Cheddar Cheese (8 oz, grated)

*What to Do*

- Mix all ingredients except lettuce together and form into patties.
- Cook over grill or in a frying pan until done.
- Serve with lettuce leaves in place of bun.

# Conclusion

Thanks for making it through to the end of *Simple Keto Cookbook* I hope, after reading Elena's story, you feel inspired to embark on your own keto journey!

Remember, when you begin your keto diet, speak to your physician first to make sure the keto diet is right for you. While the diet has been proven successful for many happy and healthy individuals worldwide, there are circumstances which might mean you would be better off to try something else. Elena's story is one of many who has found successful diet and exercise plans that worked well for them. This doesn't mean her diet and exercise plan will be exactly what you need.

If the keto diet is right for you, I hope that you will find Elena's story and recipe list to be something that will be useful to you in reaching your goal of a happy, healthier lifestyle.

The next step is to sit down and design a meal plan and exercise routine that works great for your busy lifestyle. Think about the resources available in your hometown. Like Elena, do you have a Wellness Center? Are there local gyms that work well with your work hours? Do you have parks and space at home to develop a work out routine outside of the gym?

Also, remember the tips you learned about shopping when you make your next trip to the grocery store. Keep your eye out for those tricky nutrition fact labels to ensure you know exactly what you are purchasing.

Finally, if you found this book useful in any way, a review on Amazon is always appreciated!

* 9 7 8 1 7 2 0 9 3 3 0 5 2 *